WHAT IF IT'S

RINGING IN THE EAR
TINNITUS RELIEF

SKINNY BOOK™

BY:

MURRAY GROSSAN, MD

ISBN: 978-0-9853555-5-5

Portrait Health
Publishing™

Published by Portrait Health Publishing, Inc.
175 E Hawthorn Parkway, Suite 235
Vernon Hills, IL 60061
www.portraithealthpublishing.com

Cover Design by Jeremy Shape

Disclaimer

Table of Contents

Introduction

A personal welcome to the Grossan Tinnitus Relief Program.

A. RINGING IN THE EAR *This book*
B. Ear Ringing Relief App *Available on iTunes*

When 10 million persons with Tinnitus seek relief, they may be told that nothing can be done for it, or to use "Miracle Ear Drops."

Now, the whole person program that Murray Grossan, M.D. has used effectively for his own patients is here. It is presented in a manner easy to follow, just like learning a tennis serve! Best of all, you are provided with a coach, your mirror, to show you when you do the actions right.

Relief from ear ringing requires that ALL the tinnitus factors be addressed, including full understanding (cognition), and new brain circuits. This whole body approach works, because when you understand WHY you do these actions, then the mind is engaged in the therapy.

Murray Grossan, M.D.

Dr. Grossan has published on Tinnitus therapy since 1970. He is board certified in Ear Nose and Throat, (Otolaryngology), and practices at Cedars Sinai Medical in Los Angeles.

What is Tinnitus?

Tinnitus is a condition where you hear a sound but it is not from outside the head. Instead, it is being generated inside your head, either in the ear, the hearing nerve, the connections to the brain, or the brain itself. Despite advances in medical technologies, there is no test or device available to objectively measure or definitively detect tinnitus. You can accurately measure blood pressure and see a fracture, but not tinnitus.

The prevalence rate of tinnitus is astounding. An estimated fifty million persons have tinnitus, but ten million have a symptomatic problem with it. Why this difference? Why do some persons have severe hearing loss and no tinnitus, while others with the same hearing loss have tinnitus? Why do some persons with normal hearing have tinnitus?

Let's explore the answers by first introducing key terms to understanding tinnitus.

There is *subjective tinnitus*, where only the patient can hear it.

To date, even the most advanced instruments available to us are not able to detect it.

Then, there is *objective tinnitus* in which a sound can actually be heard by the examiner and can be recorded using medical technologies. Objective tinnitus is often due to an enlarged blood vessel, an aneurism, or a muscle within the head that is repeatedly contracting, similar to an eye twitch. Objective tinnitus is rare.

Here we will discuss subjective tinnitus.

Tinnitus can also occur when a doctor cuts the auditory nerve, the main nerve from the ear to the brain, or this nerve becomes damaged due to trauma to the head. Somehow, the brain takes over to make up for the sound not coming from the ear. Subjective tinnitus is made of nerve activity of the ear, nerve, and brain. The reason it is so hard to cure is that we cannot measure it objectively or get to the very spot from which it is coming.

Tinnitus is not psychological:

Tinnitus is not a sign of mental illness, weakness, or impending serious illness. MRI scans for tinnitus show normal brain, unless a specific condition is present. It is not psychological in origin, although stress can make the symptoms worse. It can occur in persons who are kind and loving, or it can occur in persons who are lazy and mean. It can start in tall or short persons. Like a twisted ankle, it is not of psychological origin.

How do you measure tinnitus?

Your doctor will order an audiogram to see if you have a hearing loss. In a soundproof booth you will be asked to raise your finger when you hear specified sounds of varying frequencies measured on the Hertz (Hz) scale. The numbers are like the piano scale from low to high. The 500 Hz sound is like the lower or left side of the piano; the 8000 Hz is like the upper or right side of the piano keys.

Figure 1. Sample Audiogram

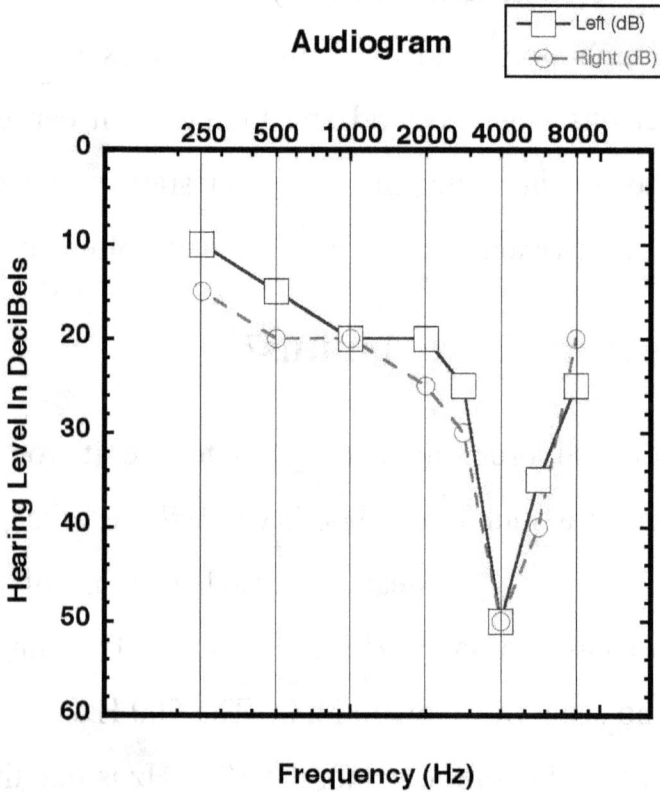

Audiogram — Left (dB), Right (dB)

X-axis: Frequency (Hz) — 250, 500, 1000, 2000, 4000, 8000
Y-axis: Hearing Level In DeciBels — 0, 10, 20, 30, 40, 50, 60

If your hearing is normal, you will hear at a 0 to 15 decibel (dB) level. Many persons are able to hear well at the 500 to 3000 tones, and then have a diminished ability to hear the higher tones of 4000 Hz to 8000 Hz.

When you are tested for tinnitus, the examiner will ask you which of the audiogram sounds resembles your own subjective tinnitus. For example, if the 6000 Hz sound resembles your tinnitus, she will record that the tinnitus matches the 6000 Hz sound. Then she will ask how loud it is by presenting the same sound to you at various volumes. For example, "His tinnitus is matched at 6000 Hz at a volume of 30 db."

In your Grossan Ear Ringing Relief App, you can play the various sounds and identify which of those matches your own tinnitus. Later I will discuss using that sound for a process called masking.

Tinnitus Q and A:

Another tinnitus measurement is a Q and A. This gives some

indication of the severity of your tinnitus, how it affects you. You are invited to take this questionnaire (see Appendix at end of this book) before starting the Grossan Ear Ringing Relief App and program. Then repeat it in three months. You can compare your score before and after. You can also repeat the test later. This can give you a measurement of your success.

Tinnitus causes:

Most commonly, tinnitus follows exposure to loud sounds that cause a hearing loss. Common causes of hearing loss include industrial noise such as jackhammer and machinery. Rock concerts and ear buds with the music playing full blast are a common problem. Shooting practice of police officers and fire engine sirens of fire fighters are frequent work-related etiologies. Certain drugs may also cause tinnitus. Metabolic and circulatory problems such as diabetes and hypertension are also known causes.

As an illustrative example, an individual with a hearing loss is tested and shown to have the poorest tone at 4000 Hz, and hearing is located; however, other nerves connect here too. If you think of this nucleus as a place where you change trains, sometimes the ticket clerk puts you on the wrong train, and instead of landing in New York, you end up in Atlanta. There are inputs into this nucleus from the jaw, neck, and face, and this explains how non-sound trauma can lead to tinnitus. Tinnitus that comes from input of muscles is called ***Somatosensory Tinnitus***. An example of this is the pain from whiplash traveling to the Dorsal Cochlear Nucleus and is misdirected to the hearing part of the brain. See Figure 2.

FIGURE 2. Pathway of Sound to the Brain

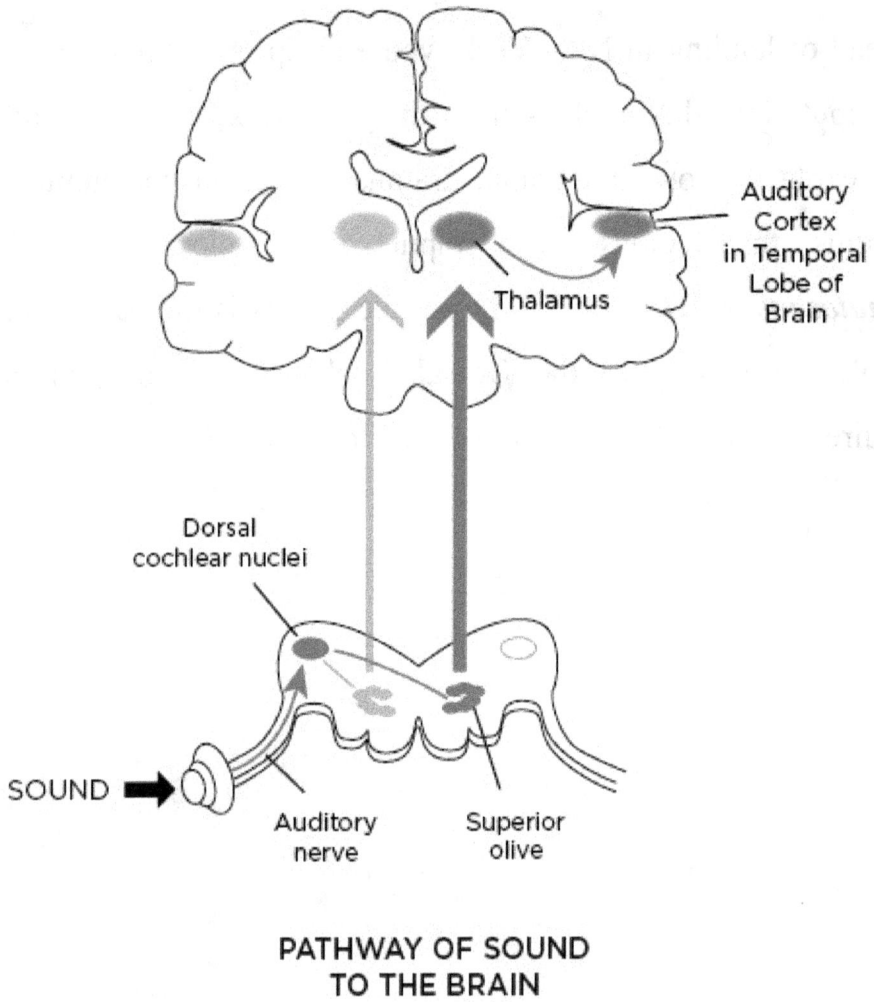

PATHWAY OF SOUND
TO THE BRAIN

With the widespread use of ear buds and mp3 players, the prevalence of tinnitus is certain to increase among all age groups, particularly when they seat the little kids in front of the blaring eight- foot speakers at the wedding. Hearing loss is the most common cause of tinnitus.

A recent article in the New York Times details how restaurants and bars are deliberately pumping in very loud music, so loud that patrons have to shout the orders in order to be heard. Because persons can't talk or relax, they finish eating soon and make room for more customers. (They also consume more food). Of course, the waiters and bartenders will end up with hearing loss and tinnitus. I advise you to download a free sound meter on your smartphone so you will know when the sound is above 85db to avoid this damaging exposure.

The Occupational Safety and Health Administration (OSHA) standard is that no worker should be exposed to 85db for more than eight hours a day.

Other causes of tinnitus:

- Outer ear: Wax or cotton against the ear drum

- Middle Ear: Fluid buildup in the middle ear

- Inner Ear: Fluid pressure in the inner ear – the cochlea. This includes conditions like Meniere's Disease, Cochlear Hydrops and problems of fluid drainage.

- Pressure or distortion of the nerves as they go to the brain can cause tinnitus.

- Changes in the fluids of the brain can cause tinnitus.

- Impulses from nerves from the jaw and neck are a factor.

- Many drugs can cause tinnitus including aspirin and the non-steroidal anti-inflammatory drugs such as Ibuprofen. If you suddenly develop tinnitus when you start a new drug, check with your doctor.

Although aspirin and related products can cause tinnitus, usually it stops when the aspirin is discontinued. The "baby dose" of aspirin (81 mg daily) that people take to prevent complications of a heart attack or stroke does not typically cause tinnitus. Most patients can continue this if they have tinnitus.

Systemic conditions such as hypertension, diabetes, and elevated cholesterol are important items to consider as causing tinnitus and hearing loss. These conditions interfere with circulation and metabolism. It is important to treat these conditions for overall health as well as to prevent hearing loss and tinnitus.

Certain tinnitus conditions are readily diagnosed and treated. In Meniere's Disease or Cochlear Hydrops, there is an excess of fluid in the inner ear. This fluid build-up is detected as part of a comprehensive hearing evaluation. Typical Meniere's disease shows hearing loss, tinnitus, dizziness and a full feeling in the ear. Where there is extra fluid in the inner ear, doctors may prescribe a special type of diuretic called a carbonic anhydrase inhibitor such as methazolamide. When there is a difference in the hearing between the two ears, doctors look for the cause. This may require an MRI to examine the hearing nerve and pathways. The MRI can detect minute changes in the hearing nerve.

Hypertension can be a cause of tinnitus that is cleared by

correcting the elevated blood pressure. Physical causes such as a concussion or whiplash may result in tinnitus. Stress by itself is not a cause of ringing in the ear, but stress may aggravate an existing tinnitus when the tinnitus sound is identified as a danger.

When you hear the tiger:

Tinnitus is actually made worse because we are born with a built-in defense against intruders. We inherit a system: when we hear the tiger's sound, to fight or flee. In tinnitus symptoms, that subjective sound is mistaken for the tiger with the corresponding fight/flight reaction. This response is fully automatic; modern man hears subjective tinnitus and responds with primitive man's tiger response.

Primitive man heard the outside twig snap and experienced an adrenalin rush. Those who had a good tiger sound response survived and we are their descendants. The goal here is to unconsciously "know" that the tinnitus is NOT a dangerous intruder, to change that reflex. However changing that inborn reflex takes some practice.

Recent studies published in Lancet[1] concluded that learning to understand comprehensively that the ringing sound is not a tiger is the best therapy. This is called Cognitive Therapy or Cognitive Behavioral Therapy and is the primary purpose of this book and the ringing in the ear app.

1. Cima RF, Maes IH, Joore MA, et al. Specialised treatment based on cognitive behaviour therapy versus usual care for tinnitus: a randomised controlled trial. Lancet. 2012;379:1951-1959.

Conditions that Make Tinnitus Worse:

Stress (fight or flight) chemicals

Anxiety reinforcement

Being told there is no treatment

Poor sleep

The Stress Response to Tinnitus

We are all born with a fight/flight reaction to noise. Primitively, almost any noise represented danger and would elicit a fight/flight response. Unfortunately, if your body misidentifies the tinnitus as a tiger or danger, then the same primitive fight/flight reaction takes place with increased heart rate, rapid breathing, tight muscles, sweating, and increased outflow of adrenalin. This stress response may be complicated by a lowered immunity, depression, fatigue and less sleep. Excess stress chemicals actually shrink the size of the hippocampus, an organ in the brain that has to do with memory. Some autoimmune diseases – psoriasis, rheumatoid arthritis and others are hypothesized to be stress related. The stress reaction amplifies the tinnitus sensation. When you hear an unknown sound, the stress reaction may be triggered automatically. When you recognize that sound as a tree branch scratching your window, then there is no stress reaction. The sooner you recognize that the tinnitus is not a tiger/threat, the fewer unwanted chemicals enter your body.

People who live around noise such as train tracks or traffic are bothered by this inborn reaction at first. Once the body recognizes it as a non–tiger, non–danger, then the stress reaction to that noise ceases. In Cognitive Therapy, patients learn that the tinnitus is not a threat. In doing so, they change the chemical reaction. I will show you how to react to tinnitus so that you avoid the unwanted chemistry.

Anxiety reinforcement:

Anxiety reinforcement can make any condition worse; the more it itches, the more nervous you get, the more you scratch, and the more it itches. Your young daughter just got her driver's license and she isn't home at ten o'clock, as scheduled. It is snowing. It is now ten-thirty. The more you worry the more stress chemicals enter your body; your pulse is faster and your blood pressure is raised.

When anxiety reinforcement complicates tinnitus, the tight muscles, neck and temporomandibular joint (TMJ) adds to the tinnitus. Everyone experiences tinnitus at some time or another. It is nearly always temporary. If the anxiety response doesn't occur, it can "go away." In medicine, we see anxiety making everyday conditions worse; the girl beginning to menstruate is assured by her loving mother and sister that this is "Okay," and is part of becoming a mature woman, has minimum symptoms all her life. The girl with the evil stepmother who screams that this is punishment for her evil thoughts has difficulties the rest of her life. Similarly, relaxing at onset sets the stage for minimal symptoms or hopefully none.

Nothing can be done for it:

If a doctor tells the patient, "There is nothing you can do for it," that is like saying the tiger is outside the cave and there is no means of escaping it. Of course, you feel distressed. Such a hopeless feeling unleashes bad chemistry. On the other hand, if someone with tinnitus is given a program to follow, this is like saying you have a shotgun and a bright flashlight to protect yourself from the tiger, and even kill it. The chemistry that you get when you take charge helps your healing. My goal is to give you a program to fix that tiger response from your tinnitus. You will have less tinnitus symptoms when you are conscious that the tinnitus is NOT a tiger, and you have a program that you can follow.

Poor Sleep:

In the 2012 Ear Nose and Throat meeting in San Diego, Dr K. Yaremchuk of Henry Ford Hospital in Detroit demonstrated that the severity of tinnitus was directly related to poor sleep. Less sleep → more tinnitus. Of course, with adrenaline flooding your body, you won't fall asleep easily.

What works for sleep:

Set the sleep clock. Go to bed at same time nightly. Wind down with a complex sleep routine: Remove cosmetics, wash face, brush hair, clean nails, cream the face and hands, warm bath or shower, etc. When there are five procedures you do routinely, your inborn sleep clock works best. For sleep, distraction by a dull familiar input helps. Music you know may make you sleepy. Sounds of a waterfall, soft music – best is Broadway musicals. TV is good – for men the shopping channel and for women the sports channel. When you have practiced the ten actions of this app program below, you will significantly improve your sleep situation. You can use the features of the app to listen to white noise.

The purpose of my program is to develop responses that will counter the factors that might make your tinnitus worse. When you practice the Grossan Ear Ringing Relief Program, you send signals to the brain and the autonomic nervous system that tells them that there is no tiger, no need for the adrenalin. You will use a visualization that puts out the healing factors. When you visualize using all your senses before the tinnitus, you get different body chemistry by adding your brain to the healing.

Summarized below is a case study of an actual patient with tinnitus and how he successfully overcame the debilitation caused by his symptoms.

Abernathy B., age thirty-eight, lived in a second floor apartment in Manhattan. He was accustomed to the traffic noise. He drove to Chicago, and on his way stopped in a small town with a very quiet motel. As he lay down to sleep he became aware of a noise in his head, a ringing. With the Manhattan noise—taxis, fire engines, etc.—he had previously not been aware of this sound. He cancelled his Chicago trip and rushed back to New York. His family doctor told him that he should see a specialist right away. It turned out that he couldn't get an appointment for a week. He stayed at home and increased his anxiety until he finally saw the doctor. Some tests were performed and after reviewing the tests, the doctor said he needed to get an MRI of the ear. That took days, and finally, two weeks after his return from the trip, he learned that tinnitus is a subjective sound, and in his case was not the sign of any disease. But this reassurance didn't help him. For two weeks he had flooded his body with chemicals of anxiety and was reinforcing his tinnitus symptoms. He had visualized the worst outcomes.

The more he identified the tinnitus as "bad," the more that was implanted into his circuits. Finally, he used the Ear Ringing Relief Program to reduce his anxiety, corrected his cognition of identifying tinnitus as "bad," and then his symptoms did improve.

The reason the Grossan Ear Ringing Relief iPhone App is successful is that in nearly every case of tinnitus, various factors contribute to the symptoms. These may include muscles of the middle ear such as the tensor tympani and stapedius, muscles of the jaw, and cervical muscles as well. See Figure 3.

The Ear Ringing Relief App is Available on iTunes.

FIGURE 3. MUSCLES OF THE MIDDLE EAR

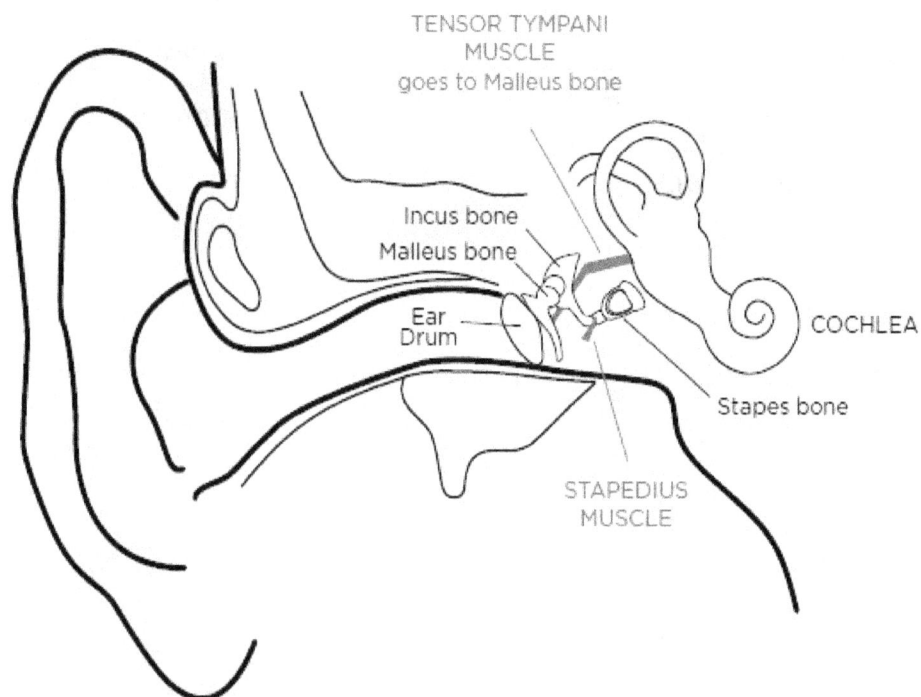

TENSOR TYMPANI
MUSCLE
goes to Malleus bone

Incus bone

Malleus bone

Ear
Drum

COCHLEA

Stapes bone

STAPEDIUS
MUSCLE

TENSOR TYMPANI MUSCLE
STAPEDIUS MUSCLE

Patients improve when any unwanted input from these areas are reduced. A useful analogy: you agree to pay for any electric bill over ten dollars. If you burn nine light bulbs, you don't have to pay. But if you burn eleven bulbs, you get a bill to pay. Similarly, if you keep the impulses from ear, jaw, neck, ear muscles below "ten", you won't generate enough "electricity" to have symptoms.

You are not just an ear. You are complex with job, kids, neighbors, etc. With my app program, I have covered actions that can account for many factors that may affect your tinnitus, for example sleep.

Let's examine the program further. The Grossan Ear Ringing Relief Program consists of ten actions that must be physically performed; reading about them won't heal you.

Measured Breathing, Mirror and Recall:

In stress, you breathe rapidly. In actions 1–3 you practice breathing so that your exhalation is longer than your inhalation.

This tells the stress center that there is no stress situation here. This stops the stress chemicals.

In stress you tighten your muscles, especially your jaw as you prepare to fight. Therefore, in actions 4, 5 and 6 you use a mirror to feedback to you if your muscles are relaxed. Originally I used special machines that fed back to the patient the amount of electricity the muscles were producing; the tighter the muscle the more the electricity. This information was fed back (biofeedback) to the patient via a large dial, so they could see that relaxation would lower the electrical output. This system is available at biofeedback clinics. Here, in this app program you use a mirror to feed back to you if your face, jaw or shoulders are tight or relaxed. Actually the mirror feedback works well. Plus you have the advantage that you can do this at home daily, and you don't have to drive downtown and pay for parking.

Actions 8 and 9 improve on overall muscle relaxation of the entire body. The relaxed muscles signal the stress center – no stress – and this stops the unwanted products.

In stress you imagine the worst outcome. In steps 7 and 10 you use all your senses to visualize and recall past good health. When you recall a fun day at the beach, before the tinnitus, you replicate that good chemistry in your body. When you recall, using all your senses, a time when you were fully relaxed, your brain/body remembers and you can relax as well.

All these actions contribute to better sleep, which aids the relief of tinnitus. We see tinnitus from tight neck muscles, tight jaw joint –TMJ, and conditions affecting middle ear muscles. What is clear is that relaxing any spasm or tightness of those muscles is helpful. When an inflamed muscle is healed, products are released into the body that helps the whole patient feel better. This is why you feel so good after a massage.

We want to make these actions fully automatic, so let's associate a color for each action.

When you see a red light, you press the brake. When you see the green light, you press the accelerator. This is fully automatic; something you developed by repetition. If I were to go into your brain and cut the connection, then you would be forced to think each time you see the red light, recognize that it is for stopping and think about finding the brake pedal and figure out how much pressure to use. Instead, it is fully automatic. When you were age fourteen, you didn't have that automatic foot to brake on red light response.

If we make these actions fully automatic, that is a huge plus. All you have to do is associate a color with the action each time you do it. After repetition, for example, when you see a green dress, your brain will automatically relax your face. That reflex bypasses your thinking brain so that it is an unconscious action. One significant advantage to these reactions being on autopilot is that the more your muscles are relaxed, the more your body can supply glycogen – the brain food – to the brain. It is not necessary to do the color association; however, for some persons it has worked fabulously. Here are the ten actions to relieve your tinnitus from the Grossan Ear Ringing Relief - Tinnitus Program.

Ten Actions for Tinnitus Relief:

1. Red. Draw your attention strongly to inhalation, using a count of four. Inhale slowly and silently count to 4. Think of oxygen going to your ear, nerve, and brain. Think of elements entering your body that will heal you.

2. Orange. Use a count of six on exhalation. Exhale slowly and silently count to 6. You want to relax as you exhale so that you don't reinforce the tinnitus. As you exhale, envision that unwanted elements are being expelled. You relax on exhaling knowing that your tinnitus will improve with a relaxed attitude.

3. Yellow. Breathe a four-count inhalation, with good oxygen coming into the hearing system, and unwanted elements going out during a six-count exhalation, with relaxation. This is therapeutic. You inhale, pause, and then exhale. Here, when you pause, you tell your body to relax because the tinnitus is not a threat. This is important because you are changing your cognition and perception as to what tinnitus is.

The actual duration of inspiring or expiring is not a factor here; don't actually time these. It is the silent counting that is important. When you focus/count this way, you are totally present.

4. Green. See your face relax in the mirror. Relaxing your face in the mirror relaxes your seventh cranial nerve, the facial nerve, which is involved with your ear, face and the stapedial muscle of the middle ear. When you pause at the end of inhalation, say to yourself that you can fully relax your face because there is no danger from the tinnitus.

Here as in actions 5 and 6 you use a mirror to feed back to yourself when you do it right. With the mirror, you can see if your face is tight; if so, relax it until you see it become relaxed. Your face sends major signals to your brain; smiling raises your immunity and you have fewer colds.

Figure 4. Use the Mirror to See the Jaw Relax

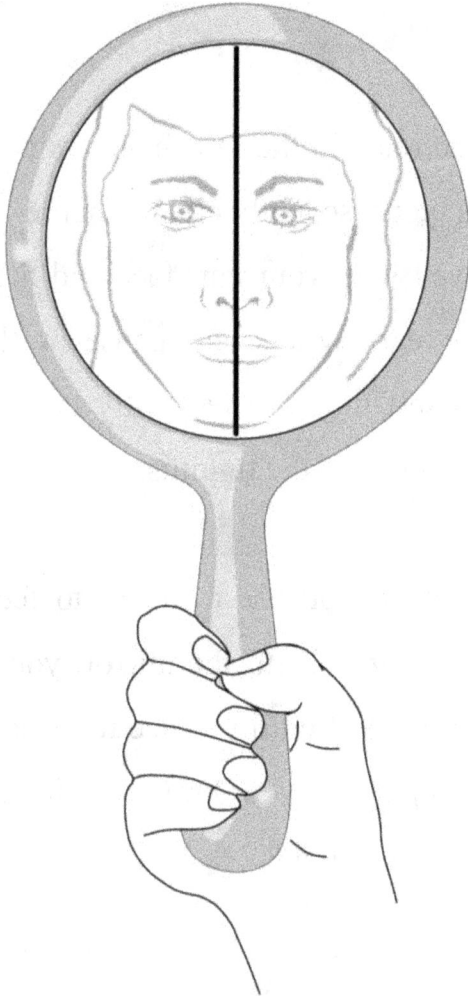

5. Blue. Relax your jaw. Use the mirror to SEE the jaw relax. The jaw can be a factor with tinnitus and relaxing it helps tinnitus. Draw a straight vertical line down the center of the mirror. Line up your face to make sure that the jaw opens in the midline. If it is not opening in the midline, practice this exercise until your muscles are balanced for the jaw and you always open in the midline. This action is also a cure for TMJ problems because when the jaw opens to the side, this means that the jaw muscles are not balanced, which may be the actual cause of the tinnitus. Here you don't deliberately open your jaw. Instead, you relax your jaw muscles so that it opens by gravity.

6. Indigo. Relax your shoulders. See your shoulders relax in the mirror. Relaxed muscles are the key to healing. Tight neck muscles can be a factor in tinnitus. Use this mirror action to relieve and release tight muscles in the neck. Relaxing your shoulders also relaxes your chest and diaphragm. Exaggerate your inhalation by raising your shoulders and see the shoulders drop on exhalation.

7. Purple. Recall a time before you had tinnitus. This directs the body to change chemistry back to before the tinnitus. Visualize with all your senses a happy time without the tinnitus. Visualize using taste, smell, sight, feel, sound a fun day at the beach. Hear the waves, taste the hot dog, feel the warm sun, smell the salt air, see the birds and people. Alternately: Visualize, recall, using all your senses being pleasantly totally and fully relaxed. The more your whole body muscles are relaxed, the less you reinforce your tinnitus.

8. White. Jacobson's progressive relaxation - the more your whole body muscles are relaxed, the less you reinforce your tinnitus. Using the counted breathing, relax from your toes to the top of your head. This system was developed in 1950 by Dr Edmund Jacobson and has been tested and proven over sixty years to relax the whole body. It is used to treat hypertension, headaches, back and neck problems related to tight muscles, as well as for overall relaxation.

9. Silver. Raise your index finger. Take three measured breaths. On the third breath, drop your finger to quash the

noise. This can be on the ear or the temple where the eighth nerve runs.

Or imagine the finger as a baton leading the orchestra. When the finger drops on the third breath the orchestra stops the sound. Use the onset of tinnitus as a signal to do the finger drop. With practice, this works for any stress situation.

Jolene had practiced action nine. She was apprehensive about her job review. When she sat down for the interview, there was a silver water pitcher on the desk, so she was fully relaxed because her action nine was automatically triggered by the silver. She could drop her finger without being noticed

10. Gold. Guided visualization using five senses

Go on an imaginary trip to a tropical forest. The sounds are muffled and there is no traffic noise. Imagine how quiet everything is, except for the patter of rain. Smell the forest, taste the fruit, see the flowers, feel the rain, hear the rain. Spend time experiencing the quiet forest and the sound of the gentle rain. You feel joy here.

Another visualization is to step into a time machine, go to a future city where they use special light beams to cure you of your tinnitus. Imagine a futuristic healing place: you hear wonderful music, you are bathed in special solutions with waves that massage you, you are given liquids to drink, and you are moved to a room with wonderful aromas. Special flickering lights are focused on various parts of your body, these feel good, like a gentle massage. After this, you feel joy at feeling great. Note: hearing, feeling, taste, smell, and sight—it is important to engage all your senses. This enables your mind to do the healing process.

Many other healing visualizations are described in my book, *Stressed? Anxiety? Your Cure is in the Mirror.* What is most important is that all the senses plus joy must be recalled.

You Need Repetition:

Reading about these ten actions has no value whatsoever, any more than reading about weightlifting builds muscles. Just as you must lift the weights, go to the gym, etc. for building muscle, so must you perform the actual actions every day to build new tracks. A minimum of ten minutes a day is needed. You can use the Ear Ringing Relief App to do the actions every hour on the hour. The App will help you to build new connections, new habits, new brain functioning. This App simply reminds you to do the actions on a daily basis; then you will build the tracks for a lifetime of better health.

Get in the habit of doing the relaxation whenever you are aware of the tinnitus. Let the tinnitus be a signal to relax, as in this program. The reason this program is so effective is that it deals with the multiple factors that may input to produce tinnitus, including impulses from neck, jaw, and middle ear muscles. More important, you are changing the body chemistry with less stress chemicals and more healing ones. With this relaxation and visualization, you actually increase benefits of the healing factors when you take vitamins and minerals that supply the known elements for good hearing and nerve function. Supplements for hearing work best when you are relaxed, when you visualize it working for you. You can do the ten actions all at once for ten minutes too: whichever works best for you. What is important is the repetition.

There is a field of therapy called Psychoneuroimmunology. They research why relaxation heals. For example, in any scientific study, a percentage of the patients get well with the good pill. But a certain percentage of patients get well with the sugar pill – the placebo. This research shows that the brain has a tremendous effect on healing of almost any condition.

This App program is based on those findings:

When you relax, your body heals better.

When you understand what the therapy is supposed to do, how it works, you heal better because your mind then aids in the healing.

If you visualize the pill / therapy working, the mind supports the healing.

To see how this works, here is an example of my typical tinnitus patient:

Bill S. age 45. Bill was stopped for traffic on a busy freeway. Suddenly he was rear- ended and his car was totaled. He developed tinnitus in his left ear, along with neck pain, and headaches. The front air bag deployed, as did the left sided one. He was referred to me eight weeks after the accident. He was receiving physical therapy. His audiogram showed reduced hearing in the left ear at 6000 Hz and tinnitus at 6000 Hz, 15 decibels below his hearing level. When I examined him, his neck was painful. He opened his jaw to the right side severely, and he couldn't sleep because of the tinnitus. I stressed the importance of actions five and six for his jaw and neck. He used step seven to recall before he had the tinnitus. He listened to his favorite music. He structured his sleep and fell asleep with the TV playing on the shopping channel. He took supplements for hearing. When he returned a month later, his symptoms were significantly improved. It is impossible to measure how much the TMJ, the neck the relaxation of the fifth and seventh nerve contributed, but why not combine this therapy since it works?

Note: Bill did develop tinnitus from the accident. But the jaw and neck contributed to the symptoms, and his anxiety had amplified his symptoms.

You often get anxiety reinforcement due to an error in cognition or perception. How do you perceive the glass of water? Is it ½ full or ½ empty?

Cognition: Eloise saw the advertisements for Shingles Vaccine. She assumed it was a sham because there were so many ads. No, I explained, getting the vaccine is needed for your health.

Cognition: She feels a lump in her breast. She asks her sister who says it must be a tumor and how terrible that she will have to have her breast removed. She reads the breast cancer information and is worried. When she sees the doctor she is reassured that it is probably just a cyst.

Such errors in cognition occur all the time, especially in tinnitus.

Cognitive therapy convinces the brain that the tinnitus sound is not a tiger, or a danger, or a bad thing. It is just like an itch or a twitch, where the nerve is discharging. It is very important to convince the brain that the tinnitus is not a threat, a growth, a disease any more than an itch is a disease to be feared. Note, you don't attack the tinnitus, you discover what it really is.

Here is an example of cognition:

The young police recruit, after shotgun practice without proper ear-muffs, complains to "Old Sarge" about having ringing in the ears. "Old Sarge" snorts, "Hey we all get that. It's 'nothin'. It comes with the job." And so the recruit doesn't amplify the condition. The tinnitus is there but it is not a stress. There is no anxiety reinforcement. But if he had been told that this might be a tumor, he might have reinforced the "bad" cognition and laid new nerve tracks that are not healthy.

Grossan Ear Relief Program for Tinnitus— Cognitive Therapy

1. Relax and inhale energizing air.

2. Exhale toxins and waste products.

3. As you breathe in to a count of four and out to a count of six, be fully relaxed because you are not in a danger mode.

4. Relax your face because there is no threat of danger. The tinnitus is simply another kind of itch.

5. Relax your jaw. There is no battle or fight coming. The tinnitus is not a threat. No, you are not going to attack the tiger with your teeth.

6. Relax your shoulders. The tinnitus is just a minor annoyance like nasal buggers.

7. Before I had tinnitus, I heard about it and it had no importance to me. Let's keep that attitude. Tinnitus is not cancer or fever or a bad smell. No one outside of me even knows I have it.

8. I can relax my whole body because there is nothing to worry or fear.

9. Whenever I pay attention to my tinnitus, I realize that it is

nothing to pay attention to, and I take three breaths, then drop my finger and squash it.

10. I envision things that tinnitus is not: it is not a car accident, it is not a knife wound, it is not a high fever, it is not a bleeding ear, it is not an amputation. It is more like a minor itch.

The cognitive program reduces the tinnitus symptom so that it is merely an annoyance like roadwork being done outside your house and can be ignored. Most important is that it is not magnified or amplified by anxiety. By changing how you perceive this subjective symptom, you react differently to it.

I live in earthquake country and you can be sure I get stressed when I feel the house shaking. But I knew that the builders were out there building a road and using large hammers that made the house shake; cognition – there was no stress.

What is Masking?

Often, covering the sound with other sounds, such as pleasant music, is beneficial. I ask my patients to have pleasant music playing in the home or on their iPod® or other personal listening device, and always at levels that permit conversations. Just as a radio will cover or mask the sound of a loud ticking clock, so will the music mask the tinnitus. But with Broadway musicals, the mind is also engaged for further distraction from the tinnitus by the words.

If there is a hearing loss that requires hearing aids, or others have commented that you are listening to the television at a loud volume, seek the evaluation of a qualified hearing professional, since hearing aids can amplify regular sounds and mask the tinnitus. A hearing aid for tinnitus works well because now familiar sounds are heard, you are no longer straining to hear, and there is better relaxation. A hearing aid is the best masker.

Masking therapy:

A form of masking is done by putting the same tinnitus sound into the affected ear. The mechanism is that the outside sound masks or inhibits the inside sound. To hear that outside sound requires a certain energy from your ear; the energy is used up listening outside and none is left over for the inside sound. Because you are hearing the outside sound, and it is just like your inside sound, therefore the inside sound isn't a "bad thing."

The Grossan Ear Ringing Relief App provides you with various sounds that are used in doing hearing tests. Sample the sounds and see which resembles your tinnitus. Then play that sound at a low volume, so that the sound is no longer coming from you. This helps your brain recognize that this sound is only a "radio sound" and not a "bad sound." As you play the sound at a low volume your body becomes accustomed to it and learns to ignore it. This principle is used in TRT or Tinnitus Retraining Therapy.

Tinnitus Inhibition:

Hearing the App sound that matches your tinnitus will inhibit your tinnitus for a period of time. For some persons, playing the masking tone from the App may inhibit the tinnitus for hours.

You no longer hear your tinnitus after listening to the outside masker. You need to try this to judge your own tinnitus inhibition following the masking. What is important is that Tinnitus Inhibition can be improved.

Angela could play her tinnitus sound from the App for 30 minutes, and then she was free of tinnitus for 15 minutes. As she practiced and visualized the improvement, after a month, listening to the masking sound for 30 minutes now inhibited her tinnitus for 60 minutes. For Roberta, the inhibition lasted most of the day.

Thus, with the low volume tinnitus sound playing constantly, you may not hear your tinnitus when you play the masking sound. Or, for example, you may play the tinnitus sound for 15 minutes and get 30 minutes with no tinnitus sound from your body.

Because you can play this masking tone any time, your body recognizes that your own tinnitus sound is not a tiger. Because the same sound is coming from the outside, your brain recognizes that the inner sound is "okay." Since the ringing is from the outside, it is not a "bad" thing.

The best masking is done when you wear a hearing aid to amplify sounds you are missing due to a hearing loss.

Nerve Enhancement:

Another method of managing tinnitus is called Nerve Enhancement, which I introduced in 1990. It is actually a form of biofeedback. First, use the Grossan Ear Ringing Relief App to identify your tinnitus sound. Now, the same tinnitus sound is played into the unaffected ear, at a low volume. Use an ear bud for this. Now use the relaxation actions. Your body now identifies the lower volume from the app. Your body is asked to adjust the volume of the actual tinnitus ear to match the app volume. Because you show the brain what the volume should be, the brain adjusts the tinnitus volume in the affected ear.

Twenty minutes a day is often effective to reduce the volume of tinnitus in the affected ear. Here the body is shown the lower volume; the body identifies it as a lowered preferred volume, the body can lower the affected ear volume to match that lower volume. When the mind is fed back the better volume from the App ear, it will lower the volume to match that App volume. Relaxing the body amplifies this effect.

New Tracks and Circuits:

You have tracks or circuits laid down that result in your tinnitus being heard. Let's lay down new tracks so that they displace the tinnitus sound. You can make your own favorite music on your iPod® or mp3 player. Record at least four hours of your favorite music. This should be familiar music that relaxes you. Example music includes Broadway Soundtracks from Sound of Music, My Fair Lady or South Pacific. (Note: these are my favorites and may not be yours). Once the music is recorded, then play this at least four hours a day. It can be background while you do other chores. It can be very soft so that you can concentrate on other tasks. What you are doing is laying down repetitive tracks that will eventually displace the "tracks" of the tinnitus. Ideally this should be recorded on an iPod® so you can do other tasks while this is playing. The more time you listen each day, the sooner the tracks will be laid down that displace the tinnitus tracks. This may take about three months to be effective. If the tinnitus is in only one ear, see if listening to it in one ear is better than listening with both ears.

Set the brakes:

I previously spoke of a braking system. Persons with normal hearing can have tinnitus. So, let's do a program where you do actions 1 through 6, in action 7 recall a time before you had tinnitus, then in action 8, go through your sound system starting with the middle ear, and mentally turn a large dial to turn off the tinnitus; the larger the imagined dial the better: fig 2

The middle ear
The inner ear
The auditory eighth nerve
The midbrain limbic system
The pathways to the brain
The temporal lobe of the brain

We need to turn off dials in each part of the hearing mechanism because today, we don't really know which system is making the tinnitus. Whether you picture this as a Mickey Mouse cartoon or some other symbolism, the brain has a special language and what works for you is probably the best way. Some persons draw a picture; some move their hands and body.

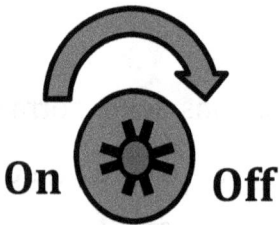

On **Off**

Or you can use a sliding scale, from loud to off

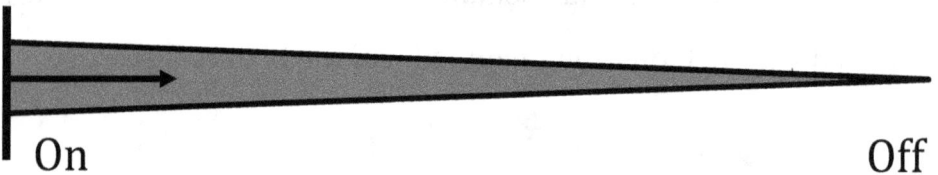

On **Off**

This may sound strange. Why would imagining a dial or on-off switch effect a change? The symbolism of the brain works in strange ways that make little sense on a conscious level. However, some of my patients have used this visualization with success.

Better Sleep:

For tinnitus relief, good sleep is very important. As previously pointed out, poor sleep directly correlates with poor tinnitus. Setting your sleep clock is so important that it is repeated here. Remember that in sleep it is necessary to set the sleep clock.

Try to go to bed daily at the same time. Wind down with a set routine of cream on the hands, brushing the hair and teeth, taking a warm bath, etc. The more steps the better, as long as they are always the same. By sticking to this routine, the sleep clock is set and you get better sleep. Many patients with tinnitus complain of not falling asleep due to their sound. An external sound generator is useful, such as the noise of a waterfall or a Broadway musical. For men, having the TV tuned to a home shopping channel, or, for women, to a sports channel, works for many because the brain is partially engaged to something dull and uninteresting. Ask your doctor if you should take a natural supplement called melatonin to help set the sleep clock. Waterfall, TV, birdsong, simple static, or favorite music, use whichever works best for you to set your sleep clock. This is repeated here because it is so important.

Tinnitus Therapy:

Various methods of tinnitus therapy are used, with varying degrees of success. Tinnitus Retraining Therapy, or TRT, teaches that the gentle sound you hear is not a tiger. This combines cognition with relaxation. Some persons respond to hypnosis. Some have found relief with acupuncture. Neuronomics is a system where altered music is listened to. By altering the tones, certain tones are stimulated. Various systems alter music so that the tinnitus sound is input: others leave the tinnitus sound out. In notched music the tinnitus sound is dropped from the music.

Recently transcranial magnetic stimulation has been used. Here, strong magnetic currents are used to alter electrical impulses in the brain.

According to a 2011 review, a few anecdotal successes have

been reported, but no complete study is available.[2]   Some patients have reported benefit from medications that relax them. The medication Xanax® has been used. Melatonin for sleep has been reported as a help.   Whichever method is being administered, when it combines cognitive therapy with reduced stress, there can be benefit.   It is important to realize that, if a hearing aid is needed to correct a hearing loss, that the rate of success for tinnitus relief is high.

2.   Meng Z, Liu S, Zheng Y, Phillips JS. Repetitive transcranial magnetic stimulation for tinnitus. Cochrane Database Syst Rev. 2011;CD007946.

Supplements:

Certain supplements such as Niacin, Serc and Gingko are directed to improve circulation. Serc is betahistine, which improves circulation to the inner ear. Although Vitamin B_{12} has been recommended for years, the results are still anecdotal.

It is reasonable to use supplements that are known to aid nerve physiology such as Pyridoxine – Vitamin B_6, Thiamine, Riboflavin and others. Recent reports did not find that Gingko was effective for relieving tinnitus [3].

In sleep apnea, tinnitus is aggravated. In laboratory studies of brain changes caused by sleep apnea, certain supplements have been found to reverse those changes; therefore these have been included in my supplement product EarAid™.

Currently Mayo Clinic is conducting a study of Magnesium

---

3. http://www.nlm.nih.gov/medlineplus/druginfo/natural/333.html. Accessed 10/23/2012.

supplement for tinnitus. This is based on evidence of its effect on nerve function. Magnesium is recommended for restless leg syndrome, which is associated with sleep disorder. At our current stage of understanding tinnitus, it is not possible to determine which supplement, whether it is Alpha Lipoic Acid, or Acetyl L Carnitine, or others might be the best therapy. Therefore these are combined so that the combination will amplify their effect. See details at (www.earaid.info).

When you visualize using all your senses at a time before the tinnitus, you are replicating the chemistry that your body had.
To help with that visualization, when you take a supplement, visualize how it works and how it will help your hearing mechanism.   Having the elements used for hearing available may aid that visualization to stop the tinnitus. Some persons will benefit, for example, by taking Alpha Lipoic Acid. The effect is further amplified if you visualize how each one works and use your brainpower to "see" it working for you. Medication enhancement is used to amplify the beneficial effects of any product you take. In medication enhancement you understand why the therapy works, visualize it actually

working, and visualize a good result. This brings your brain into the healing. You are utilizing the mechanism of engaging your whole body in the healing.

For example: Alpha Lipoic Acid:

Alpha Lipoic Acid protects against free-radical damage, supports nerve system function, and plays an essential role in generating mitochondria in the hair cells of the inner ear

Neuroplasticity and Fixing the Brain:

In my program, I use the principles of Neuroplasticity. When one part of your brain is damaged, with training, another part of your brain can take up that function. This happens when persons with stroke lose their speech. The MRI shows that the speech center no longer gets circulation. Later, after therapy, the patient has regained speech. The MRI shows a new part of the brain is doing the speech! This happened to Gabrielle Giffords where the bullet destroyed some parts of her brain. With rehabilitation and exercises, she regained most of her previous function.

In this program, we are using the principle of Neuroplasticity to have your brain develop new pathways that reduce or stop the tinnitus, and to develop a new braking system. The new pathways displace the unwanted ones. It is very important to know that in Gabrielle Giffords' therapy she was taught relaxation. That relaxation accelerated her therapy significantly. In the Grossan Ear Ringing Relief App Program you are given the tools for relaxation to speed your healing.

Laughter and smiling also use the principles of Psycho-neuroimmunology. This field examines how laughter, smiling, relaxation and visualization work. Researchers have found that immune healing factors increase with muscle relaxation, mental relaxation, favorable outlook, and smiling. They identify the actual body chemistry that changes when you stop the stress chemicals. They show how the immunity in improved when stress is reduced. These are the principles of the ten actions you will be practicing here. Why is smiling so important? Research shows that facial muscles send messages to the brain directly.

When Norman Cousins lay dying at UCLA hospital, none of

the medications had helped him. His friends brought in a movie projector and had him watch old comedies. He laughed and got well. Psychoneuroimmunology examines those chemical changes and explains the good chemistry that laughter makes.

Numerous studies show that for any illness, any condition, you heal better when you are personally engaged in getting well. When you do the ten actions daily for tinnitus relief, you certainly are fully engaged and you are using your whole body for relief.

Somatosensory Tinnitus :

Somatosensory tinnitus is a subjective tinnitus that arises from neck and jaw trauma. For some time we have known that stimulation from the neck or the TMJ - the temporomandibular joint can cause tinnitus. Indeed, after a whiplash or cervical neck injury, tinnitus may occur and disappear when the neck heals. This is why therapy for the neck is urgent when tinnitus begins after neck trauma.

Bruxism refers to persons who grind their teeth and keep the upper and lower jaws tightly clenched. This affects the muscle of the middle ear, as well as linking up with the course of the hearing circuit. For my patients, the ten actions, particularly action five, relaxing the jaw in the mirror has been effective.

There is a circuit that goes from the nerve nuclei of the neck to the dorsal cochlear nucleus of the ear mechanism and can generate tinnitus. (Refer back to Figure 2 to see this circuit illustrated). Tinnitus can also come from the temporo-mandibular joint (TMJ) and is corrected when the TMJ is corrected.

For tinnitus, it is important to do actions 5 and 6 of the Grossan Ear Ringing Relief Program to relax the jaw and shoulders and thereby get the neck relaxed. In any case of tinnitus it is important to reduce any input from these conditions that may affect the tinnitus; actions 4,5, and 6 perform this function.

TMJD –Temporomandibular Jaw Disorder:

Do you have TMJD? Look in the mirror. Draw a straight vertical line on the mirror to see if your jaw deviates. Let your jaw relax and let it fall open. Place your finger just in front of your ear canal. Do you feel a grating when you chew? Is there any pain when you press? Do you hear cracking? If you do, you may have TMJD and need to do the ten actions for relief.

Jim S. came to see me because he had pain in his left ear. He had seen his regular doctor who told him there was no infection in his ear. When he opened his mouth, his jaw deviated severely to the right. When I palpated in front of his ear canal, the actual jaw joint was tender. When he opened and closed his mouth, I could feel the noise from his jaw called crepitus. I explained about using mirror biofeedback in step five; to draw a straight line on the mirror to make sure the jaw relaxes and opens in the midline in order to balance his muscles. When I mentioned that this is also a treatment for tinnitus he volunteered that he also had tinnitus in the left ear; he hadn't mentioned it because he understood that there was no treatment for this. Jim had TMJD Temporomandibular Joint Disease. Jim practiced the mirror biofeedback and got better.

No doubt you are familiar with Pavlov's dog experiments. When the dog heard the bell, he would salivate. Just as we use a color clue to automatically do the relaxation actions, from now on, when you hear your tinnitus, let that be a signal to do the Grossan Ear Ringing Relief Program. Pick a single color of a significant action and be sure to perform that action when you see that color.

Please remember that your tinnitus will not clear in one or two days of doing the Program. It takes repetition for the Program to work, just as it does to build up a muscle. When you learn a tennis serve, you require daily repeated practice. You do better if you have a coach. With the Grossan Ear Ringing Relief Program, you have a coach – your mirror. Like the tennis serve, you need daily practice to build the new tracks.

Below is another case account of how patients affected by tinnitus are successfully using this program to relieve their tinnitus.

Marjorie, age thirty-eight, had been a rock music fan and had purchased the best seats - directly in front of the loud speakers. Now she had a high-tone hearing loss and tinnitus that matched a four-thousand tone (4000 Hz) hearing loss. She performed the ten actions of the Grossan Ear Ringing Relief Program faithfully and found that the finger as a baton in step nine gave her a sense of control, and she used this often. She would wear silver jewelry or shoes to reinforce action 9. She found that the more she practiced this, the more effective it became. Her friend, Jeremiah, had been a rock musician, but quit because of his tinnitus and hearing loss. He found that using tinnitus, as a signal to breathe relaxed was most effective. He stressed two colors, red and green, as his triggers and found that to be most effective.

Hyperacusis:

In hyperacusis, a simple sound seems uncomfortably loud, even painful. Ordinary restaurant chatter is so disturbing that persons with hyperacusis can no longer enter a crowded restaurant because the noise is too painful. There is no objective way to measure this. We are not sure what causes hyperacusis. One theory is that some part of the brain has a brake function that lowers or cuts off loud sound. Another explanation is that the tensor tympani muscle (refer back to Figure 3) is not splinting the eardrum when there are loud sounds.

For example, the artillery officer orders the large gun to be fired. His braking part of the brain signals the muscles of the middle ear to tighten up in order to reduce the vibration of the eardrum. If the tensor tympani muscle is not splinting the eardrum in noise, that can be a reason for ordinary sounds being perceived as too loud. A test called a Tympanogram can objectify this. Patients often state that they would prefer deafness to hyperacusis. In deafness, it is quiet. In hyperacusis you are bombarded with sounds that are ordinary, but they seem too loud. This condition can be associated with a hearing loss, and that makes fitting a hearing aid difficult. With neuroplasticity, we can get another part of the brain to do the braking for patients with hyperacusis.

Paul K., age thirty-one, suffered a loud industrial explosion combined with a cerebral concussion. He struck his right ear forcibly against a steel cabinet. He developed some right-sided hearing loss, as well as an annoying tinnitus. The audiologist referred him to me. She explained that he could be fitted with a hearing aid, which would restore his hearing and thereby mask his tinnitus. But the problem was, he had developed a sensitivity to loud sounds. Car horns, telephone ringing, a door slamming - all these were painful to him. By using a hearing aid, softer sounds now became much too loud, so he couldn't wear a hearing aid. He had hyperacusis. He had been through Prozac® and Xanax® to control his anxiety, but insisted that as long as there was no excess noise he was fine. He didn't see taking the drugs "when he himself wasn't crazy."

We put him on the Grossan Ear Ringing Relief Program with

emphasis on general relaxation, during which time he listened to music. Gradually, he increased the volume of pleasant music during a ten-minute session, twice daily. Slowly, he continued to increase the volume until it was actually loud. At the same time, he took the hearing supplements to supply any enzyme or vitamin needs. He improved. He couldn't return to going to rock concerts, but there was enough improvement to lead an otherwise normal life. By making the adjustments under good relaxation, he fixed the brakes and the malfunctioning part of his brain to work correctly. Now he was able to use a hearing aid successfully. Because he was relaxed as he increased the volume of the music, his brain no longer identified loud sounds as "bad."

A biofeedback method is to record a pleasant sound or music and play it in the normal ear. Gradually increase the volume. This "tells" the affected ear that this volume is OK. Then, try to play that same volume in the affected ear. The affected ear will try to do what the normal ear did. In some cases of hyperacusis, there is a failure of the tensor tympani muscle to splint the eardrum around loud sounds. Performing these actions helps improve that muscle function.

Have you ever felt and heard a fluttering in your ear and wondered if there was a fly in your ear canal? Without the fly, this is due to tensor tympani muscle spasm.

Tensor Tympani Muscle Spasm:

This is a most disturbing condition. You feel a fluttering in the ear, as though a live fly was there. There is no way for you to ignore the repeated fluttering. What makes it worse, is that you can't see into your ear canal. However, when you see the doctor she says she can't see any disease!

Sometimes these patients are incorrectly put on anxiety medication for treatment. The best treatment following an accurate diagnosis is a mirror and the Grossan Ear Ringing Relief Program.

The Tensor Tympani Muscle is located in the middle ear (Figure 3). It serves to tighten the eardrum to prevent excess movement when you anticipate a loud sound. From the name you can tell this muscle serves to splint or hold the eardrum from excess vibration. Sometimes the tensor tympani goes into spasm, similar to your eye twitching. This is an objective tinnitus and can be recorded and measured. Fortunately, the cure is fairly simple. Ordinarily, we place Electromyography (EMG) sensors on the forehead and ask the patient to reduce that electrical output. This is because the nerve that goes to the tensor muscle is best affected by relaxing the face. By reducing this electrical output, by biofeedback, you also reduce the electrical output of the tensor muscle. With the mirror you can do the same thing by using relaxed breathing and concentrating on relaxing your facial muscles, steps 1 through 6 in the Grossan Ear Ringing Relief Program. Below are two real case reports from patients who sought my assistance for a "fly in the ear."

Patrick S. had asked for an appointment as early as possible, as he was in extreme distress. No, he didn't have a fever or a real pain. He saw me because after he received a blow to his head, he developed this uncomfortable fluttering in his left ear, like a fly in the ear. He had a doctor look in his ear for a live fly. When I examined him, I explained that he didn't have any infection. I explained that he had a muscle - the tensor tympani - that normally steadies the eardrum so that when a very loud sound is anticipated or heard, it tightens the eardrum in order to avoid excess drum vibration, which could harm the hearing. Much like a twitchy eye, this muscle was contracting when there was no reason to contract; hence, the "fly in the ear" sensation. Patrick seemed to understand this mechanism pretty well, so I thought he would be successful using actions 1 through 6 of the Grossan Ear Ringing Relief Program.

Actions Program for Tensor Tympani Spasm – fifth nerve

1. Red. Count four for inhalation.

2. Orange. Count six for exhalation

3. Yellow—Practice breathing in to a count of four, then breathe out for a count of six.

4. Green. Wrinkle your face and smile to study the facial movements. Try to contract right and left sides separately. Now, concentrate on relaxing all the facial muscles as you relax

on exhalation. Mentally divide the face into three regions—upper above the eyes, middle below the eyes, and lower third below the mouth. After a minute or two, turn the face slightly to the right and relax that area in front of the ear and the ear itself.

5.Blue. Relax the jaw to reinforce the facial relaxation.

6.Indigo. Relax the shoulders to signal the ear muscles to relax.

Patrick's ear flutter stopped in two days by using this exercise. When he relaxed his facial muscles using the mirror as a biofeedback system, he was also relaxing that ear muscle.

Remember, Patrick received cognitive therapy. He now knew that this flutter In the ear was not "bad". He saw a picture of the muscle and now understood what it looked like, what it did and why it was bothering him. Once he had this knowledge he could take charge. It is possible that just knowing, "cognition", might have been enough for a cure.

Mrs. Sylvia T., age forty-seven, called and pleaded for a same-day appointment. She refused to fill out the patient form as to why she was seeing me. Finally, she told me, with considerable embarrassment, that there was a fly in her ear canal, which meant to her that she was some kind of dirty, unwashed person. When I explained to her that she had tensor tympani spasm, she was delighted that it had nothing to do with her cleanliness. Just knowing what the condition was enabled Mrs. Sylvia to get relief, she didn't require further therapy.

This condition can be objectified by using a Tympanometer, a device that records the movement of the eardrum and it shows up on a graph. In my experience, "stress" does not cause this condition, and the patient is justified in being anxious until reassured that there is no insect in the ear. On an interesting note, insects do get in the ear, and I have had my share of removing them.

Fortunately, the patients I have treated for tensor tympani muscle spasm have responded very quickly to biofeedback as part of the Grossan Ear Ringing Relief Program. They SEE how to relax the facial muscles, and that relaxation works for the tensor tympani and stapedial muscles as well.

Conclusion

In the Summer 2012 issue of *Hearing Health*, Dr. Yong Bing Shi, M.D., Ph.D. of the Oregon Health and Research Institute, evaluated the various forms of tinnitus treatment in his article, Testing Tinnitus Treatment[4]. He concludes that management of tinnitus requires a combination of various measures including better sleep and reducing stress and anxiety. In a recent edition of Lancet[5], Cima and colleagues report a controlled trial of various treatments of tinnitus at the Maastricht University in the Netherlands. They report on some 492 patients that Cognitive Therapy (cognitive behavioral therapy) gave the best results, and the longest lasting results.

Thus, the Grossan Ear Ringing Relief App includes methods that are known to help, and I have explained why they work.

---

4. Shi Y. Testing Tinnitus Treatment. Hearing Health. Vol 28 No 3 Summer 2012.

5. Cima RF, Maes IH, Joore MA, et al. Specialised treatment based on cognitive behaviour therapy versus usual care for tinnitus: a randomised controlled trial. Lancet. 2012;379:1951-1959

They can be tailored to the individual for daily use.

Sometimes a patient with tinnitus is told, "Nothing can be done for it. Learn to live with it." As you can see from this book, that is the farthest thing from the truth. Any condition can be improved when a patient takes charge and does the therapy. When you use these tools you will be bringing into full force the known factors of healing and health. I wish this works for you, as well as it has for my patients.

Tinnitus Q and A

Name

Date

Tinnitus Score: Please rate all questions on a scale from 1 – 5.

0 – Never at all   3 – It is a mild problem

1 – Slight or Occasional   4 – It is definitely a problem

2 – It is sometimes a problem 5 – It is a severe problem occurring all the time

1	Because of your tinnitus, is it hard to concentrate?	0 1 2 3 4 5
2	Does tinnitus interfere with your sleep?	0 1 2 3 4 5
3	Does the loudness of your tinnitus make it difficult for you to hear people?	0 1 2 3 4 5
4	Does your tinnitus make you angry?	0 1 2 3 4 5
5	Because of your tinnitus, do you feel desperate?	0 1 2 3 4 5
6	Do you have trouble falling sleep at night?	0 1 2 3 4 5
7	Does your tinnitus interfere with your social life (restaurants, movies, parties?)	0 1 2 3 4 5
8	Because of your tinnitus, do you feel frustrated?	0 1 2 3 4 5
9	Does your tinnitus make it difficult for you to enjoy everyday life activities?	0 1 2 3 4 5
10	Does your tinnitus interfere with your job?	0 1 2 3 4 5

11	Because of your tinnitus, are you often irritable?	0 1 2 3 4 5
12	Because of your tinnitus, is it hard to read?	0 1 2 3 4 5
13	Because of your tinnitus, do you often feel tired?	0 1 2 3 4 5
14	Because of your tinnitus, have you sought or taken antidepressant medication?	0 1 2 3 4 5
15	Because of your tinnitus, do you feel anxious?	0 1 2 3 4 5
16	Does your tinnitus get worse under stress?	0 1 2 3 4 5
17	Is it difficult to turn you attention away from your tinnitus for games or recreation?	0 1 2 3 4 5
18	Does your tinnitus make you upset?	0 1 2 3 4 5
19	Does your tinnitus control you?	0 1 2 3 4 5
20	Does your tinnitus bother you even when you are relaxed, even with relaxed breathing and thinking?	0 1 2 3 4 5

Total Score _____

After you have used the Grossan Ear Ringing Relief App for 3 months, please repeat the test to evaluate your improvement. We would love to hear from you.

Murray Grossan, M.D.